KARLA SCHUNN

TODDLER DISCIPLINE

**The Essential Guide on How to Teach The Right Values
To Your Child, Learn Different Practices and Strategies on
How to Raise Smart and Well-Behaved Kids**

Descrierea CIP a Bibliotecii Naționale a României
KARLA SCHUNN
   TODDLER DISCIPLINE. The Essential Guide on How to
Teach The Right Values To Your Child, Learn Different
Practices and Strategies on How to Raise Smart and Well-
Behaved Kids / Karla Schunn. – Bucharest: Editura My Ebook, 2020
   ISBN

KARLA SCHUNN

TODDLER DISCIPLINE

**The Essential Guide on How to Teach The Right Values
To Your Child, Learn Different Practices and Strategies on
How to Raise Smart and Well-Behaved Kids**

My Ebook Publishing House
Bucharest, 2020

CONTENTS

WHAT IS PARENTAL CONTROL?

Parental control is a term that is used to describe the watchful eye that you can have on your child while they are online when you are not around. These controls allow the parent, who holds a master account with their internet service provider, to take control over their specific allowances to the child. For many parents, this allows them some level of protection for when the child is online. Since more and more children at younger ages are getting online, the need is growing and very important is this control.

The Need

The need for parental controls is high. With many of today's pedophiles and criminals lurking online to do their dirty work, your child is at risk. You could just prohibit them from getting onto the web, but that really is not realistic anymore. The fact is that students use the internet to research their homework, to talk with their friends and to play educational (or not so educational) games online. The likelihood of taking this away from them is not high simple because much of life also revolves around being online. They shop online, they meet people online, and they need to be able to use it as a tool to aid them in many functions of everyday life.

Enter Parental Controls

As you can see, there is little hope that you will actually be able to never allow your child to get on the web. But, parental controls can help you nonetheless. With these tools, your child can safely do the things that they want while you control where they go and what they do, to a certain level. Parental controls can also help you to parent your child's use of the internet, but allowing you to set time limits and to keep them within certain websites.

Parental controls are a tool that every parent should have on their hands. Most internet service providers do offer some level of protection for your child, if you allow them their own screen name and access to the web. With the help of parental controls, you allow your child to do the things he or she needs and wants to do but to do those things safely. That's really the important aspect to remember.

PARENTAL CONTROL:
PROTECT YOUR CHILD AND COMPUTER

Parental controls allow you to keep track of what your child is doing online. Although the best case scenario is that you will be able to sit with your child and do what they need to on the web with them, this is not even remotely possible in most cases. There are many things that you can do to help protect them including using parental controls. But, these controls don't only help protect your child. Many of them can help to protect your computer and network, too. That makes them even more important for you to consider.

Protection For Your Child

The reason to use parental controls starts with the ability to protect your child. There is no doubt that this is the real reason you'll use them in the first place. The fact is that protecting your child with these tools helps to keep them out of the hands of predators that are lurking on the web. While you can't take the internet away from them always, you can protect them by using these controls to limit who they talk to, where they go online, and even how long they are online.

Parental Controls For Your Computer's Protection

In addition to providing protection for your child, parental controls also help you by protecting your overall well being including your computer's well being. For example, many parental controls provide protection from downloads. Your child isn't able to download something off the web unless you approve it. This is a very important tool as it helps to keep spyware, adware, and viruses off your computer. In addition, it will keep your child from visiting websites that have this potentially troublesome files and elements on them. That means it protect your computer as well as your child.

Parental controls have the foundation of helping your family to remain safe. You'll find many different ways to use them to safe guard your family, in fact. Take a few minutes to find out what parental controls can offer to your needs and then get them on your computer to keep your child and your computer from becoming vulnerable to what's lurking on the internet. Without you realizing it, you could be saving yourself from countless problems down the road by just setting up parental controls.

PARENTAL CONTROL: IS IT ENOUGH?

You may have seen an advertisement for parental controls. You may even be considering the purchase of this type of software. What you should realize, then, is that parental controls are only one step in the process of protecting your child. Although it seems like the solution you need, parental controls can also be one of the most important tools for your child but it may not be the only tool that is necessary.

Most parents realize the importance of monitoring their child online. But, even though you are providing this through the use of parental controls, you also need to educate your child regarding the dangers that are lurking online that allow them to be vulnerable. The fact is that many children, even younger ones, are able to navigate around the protections you put in place for them. If they do this, you may not know its happening and your child is left just as vulnerable as they were in the first place.

For that reason, education is one of the most important considerations you should have.

Educating your child about the safety necessaries online is a must. Children can easily be taught how to stay safe online, just as you teach them to stay safe in public. You just need to communicate with them what the risks are as well as how to avoid becoming a victim to these risks.

When you couple educating your child about the risks and the parental controls that you put in place, your child can and will be protected when they are online. With these controls in place, you can safely make decisions regarding the well being of your child. Without them, your child is at risk for countless online experiences. Protecting your child means educating them, as well as yourself, with the risks that are lurking.

USING PARENTAL CONTROL WISELY

Parental controls allow you, as a parent or guardian to be able to control the computer in which your child or younger adult is using. You know the importance of doing so. Online predators are out there and they are readily stalking even the youngest of children that venture onto the web. Using parental controls allows you to keep control of the situation so that you can make decisions for your child that will ultimately help them deal with what happens online.

What Can Be Done?

Each internet service provider will have their own different set of parental controls that you can use. The first thing that you will need to do is to find out what types of software are being offered to you through your provider. If you do find that these parental controls are not enough to really protect your child, you can find others available to you to purchase. Before you make that investment, remember that some internet service providers do provide this, or at least some parental controls, with their service to you.

There are many different options that you can use. Here are a few of the services that are available.

- Monitor who can send your child email.
- Monitor who your child can send emails to, as well.
- Determine who can send instant messages to your child or who your child can chat with in chat rooms. Limit them by name or age, or just allow certain ones.
- Monitor the time that they are online. Set a timer for each visit as to how much time they can be online each time they come onto the web.
- Determine which websites your child can go to as well as what type of website it is. Some limit the child to only those websites that are approved by you.

There are other services that you can use when it comes to parental controls. There is no doubt that you'll be able to find the right type of control for your needs either with your current internet service provider or with additional software that you purchase. The goal here is to find the product that offers you the overall best solution and protection for your child. This isn't the type of thing that you should put aside and do later.

ONLINE TIMERS AND PARENTAL CONTROL

With parental controls, you stay in control of what your child does online as well as what how long they are online in the first place. One of the tools that many internet service providers provide to you is that of an online timer. This timer is a tool that you should consider for a number of reasons. In many cases, it is a helpful tool that monitors how long your child has been online as well as enforces the limit that you place on that amount of time. You make the decisions and you get to keep those rules going, too.

Face it. You simply can not monitor your teen online all day every day. If you aren't home and they are online, they may be there the entire time. The internet is full of things to do, websites to visit and lots of people to interact with. It can become a very easy way to push away the time without even knowing that you are doing it. The internet does draw in children of all ages, but remember, your parental controls are in place to help provide you with the protection you need.

An online timer is a simple enough program. All you need to do is to simply tell it just how long you will allow your child to be online. There are several types of settings that you can select from, in most cases. You can choose to limit how much time your child goes online each time they do get online. Or, you can determine how many hours they can be online for each day and limit them. In addition, you can even limit how many times they can be online during the course of a week, if you like. You can limit the number of times that your child can get on the web as well as how long they are allowed to stay there.

You determine how much time your child gets online. Once you set this number, when their time is up, the software or internet service provider tells them so. If they don't sign off themselves, the provider will do it for them, helping you to enforce the rules that you've set in place. In most cases, this is a free service as part of the software you purchased. If it isn't provided, then get it and start giving yourself an extra hand of protection even when you are not home.

PARENTAL CONTROL THAT EXTENDS BEYOND YOUR INTERNET SERVICE PROVIDER

Did you know that kids are crafty creatures? You may think you have them protected online with the use of parental controls. You've done a good job at making sure that the controls are fair but that they are in place to help your child to do well throughout their time online. Most importantly, you believe your child is safe now that they are online and using the web. The problem is that your child may know a way to getting around those controls and therefore may be able to actually avoid doing so.

How Your Child Can Get Around Your Control

Teens are especially crafty, but don't put it past your older child to do this as well. The fact is that children learn things about how to do what they want to do online whether its at school or just through friends. It happens and you shouldn't believe your child is protected when he or she may not be.

What happens is simple. While your parental controls may work for your internet service provider, you child may be using another software that's already installed on your computer to get around them. What's more is that their other electronic software may also contain the ability to get online without you even realizing it. Such programs as Internet Explorer, Netscape and others are one of the easiest ways to get around parental controls. Other elements such as instant messaging that is done outside of the internet service provider, such as with a different program, chat rooms, forums and even file sharing programs are out there. What's more is that their handheld gaming systems are now able to get online in some cases.

There Is Hope, Though

The good news is that there are parental control products on the market that can still protect you from many of these services. The first thing to do is to learn what opportunities your child has to get online around your internet service provider. Find out how they are getting online simply by watching or talking to them. Then, look for the right product on the market that will help you to limit their access to the internet across all boards. You may be one of the lucky ones that has an internet service provider that actually provides this type of protection to your child through their service. If not, find out how these parental controls work and use them.

PARENTAL CONTROL: SHOULD I CREATE
A SCREEN NAME FOR MY CHILD?

Considering parental controls for your child is something all parents today that have a computer within their home should do. Here's why. Your child gets online and visits with a simple and seemingly safe online environment such as a chat room or a message board. They begin communicating with people from in their neighborhood or around the world. But, although they are just talking and being innocent, the other person that they could be talking to is nothing like what they seem. They could be a predator. Or, they could be another kid just like your own.

The problem is that there is no way of knowing who they are.

The problem with using parent controls for your child on your own screen name means that you'll have to implement those controls on yourself. This is difficult to do since most adults don't want to be limited in where they go and what they do. That's fine because many internet service providers actually allow you to create additional screen names that fit under your account. That means that you can create a new screen name for your child that can have its own parental controls on it, helping to protect your child.

Once you have your own child set up with their own screen name, the process of setting up parental controls is simple. It takes just a few minutes to go in and create the rules that you want your child following. Selecting the appropriate tools will help you to monitor what your child is doing so that you don't have to limit your own access to the internet. In most cases, different levels of protection are available so that you can select the one that's right for your child. Take the time to insure that you talk to them about why you are using parental controls. Don't use it as a punishment, but a protection for your child's well being.

Parental controls can be very limiting and they can be quite liberal. As a child gets older, he or she may not require as much protection as they did in the beginning. As a parent, it is important to educate you're your child the risks of being online. Its also important to monitor how well their parental controls are working for both your needs of protection and their needs to be online.

The right decisions can be made so that everyone can get online and do what they need and want to.

PARENTAL CONTROL: A CHILD'S VIEW

As a good parent, you realize the importance of using parental controls to help protect your child while they are on the internet. But, controlling your child's behavior online can be somewhat of a downer for them. After all, they want to get online to play fun games, to talk with their friends and yes, even to study. There doesn't have to be a limit to either side of this coin. You can set your child's parental control levels appropriately to allow them to do age appropriate things that they want to do and still have some control over the situation. But, to make this work, you have to communicate them.

Communicate Your Needs

The first thing that you should do before ever allowing your child to get online, is talk to them about the risks. If you taught your child never to talk to strangers when walking home from school and to hold an adults hand to cross the street, then you need to help them to understand the reasons why they need to be protected online as well. Simply educating them about what the risks are will provide a level of protection to your child in and of itself. But, it is up to you to make this happen for your child.

Talk to your child about internet predators. Inform your child how easy it is for an adult to pretend to be another kid. They often spend hours studying how to do this, in fact, so that they are knowledgeable of the latest trends. The end result is that your child really does believe there is another child on the other end of that instant message and they are more than willing to tell that child anything they need to know.

Talk to your child about

- What information shouldn't be given over the internet such as last names, addresses, and phone numbers.
- Tell your child never to talk about the specific school that they go to
- Talk to your child about the appropriate and inappropriate subjects that should be talked about online
- Inform your child how to react and what to do when they don't feel comfortable anymore. Make sure they know that you won't be mad at them.

- Talk to them about parental controls that are a tool you'll be using to protect them, not to limit them.

These are just a few of the very important things you need to talk to your child about in regards to getting on the web. Most children today are educated enough in computer lingo and methods to be able to get around some of the controls you put in place. For that reason, educating your child to the "why" is essential to their well being. Again, if you taught your child to never talk to strangers, you need to help them realize that the web is full of strangers.

PARENTAL CONTROL:
DIFFERENT LEVELS OF PROTECTION

With parental controls, you have the ability to keep your child safe online. These tools keep a watchful eye on your child while they are online and doing the things that they want to do there. The good news is that thee are many levels of protection in place for you to use. That means that you'll be able to successfully implement the right level of control for your child, instead of just restricting them completely. With a good internet service provider's parental controls, or outside software that you purchase, you can keep your child safe but still provide them with the ability to do what they need online.

What Levels Are Out There?

It's important to realize that there are different levels of parental controls available to you. You'll find a number of different ways to protect your child at different age levels or different skill levels. Here are a few options that may be available to you.

- **General**: This type of parental control is not limiting. It is the standard service that you, as an adult would use. It allows for free access to the internet without any restrictions in place.

- **Teens**: The next level down is that that may be more appropriate for a teenager. It restricts various elements but it does allow them to visit more freely online. It helps to control such things as pornographic websites and other potentially threatening situations.

- **Young Teens**: With a bit more protection, your pre teen or young teenager can have more access to the things that they want to do but still be protected from chat rooms that are not child specific.

- **Kids**: The lowest levels of protection come into play for those under the pre teen years. Many of the parental controls at this level protect your child from moving outside the designated areas for them. Many internet service providers offer unique online experiences geared towards these children that is completely kid only.

Parental controls are up to you to select. Don't make the mistake of thinking that your child will be happy with a kid's only area if they are a young teen. The good news is that you can find the right solution for your child and have a successful online experience that's safe, too.

WHAT CAN PARENTAL CONTROL LIMIT?

One of the first question that you as a parent needs to ask about parental controls is just what do they limit and how do they do just that. There are many different ways that predators can come into contact with your child. You need to use parental controls as well as education to help protect them from all areas in which they are vulnerable. Think of it in other instances.

You probably taught your child a secret, family password that was put in place to allow an adult other than you to pick up your child with. But, that level of protection doesn't protect them from strangers that approach them walking home from school. Parental controls must cover all areas of vulnerability.

Areas Your Child Needs Protection

Here are a few of the most important ways that you need to protect your child when they are online. Remember, this isn't everything and with new technologies as well as new ways to meet others online happening every day, you still need to monitor other areas as well.

- **Chatting**: Chat rooms are a common thing online. There are those chat rooms set up for children as young as ten to talk about games and school. Your parental controls should allow for some protection from chat rooms that aren't approved by you or aren't known to be kid safe areas.

- **Email**: Email addresses can easily be obtained. It only takes the right words in an e-mail's subject line to get your child to open on the email and get into trouble. Parental controls can limit who can send email to your child.

- **The Web**: The web browsing abilities that your child has are also important. Parental controls must protect your child from visiting websites that are not appropriate or ones that you specifically block.

- **Instant Messaging or IM's**: One of the most common ways to chat online today is through instant messaging. It's private and easy to use. Parental controls can help block unwanted individuals from chatting with your child.

All of these parental controls can be adjusted to fit your child's needs, age and your preferences. Consider limiting all of the options to fit your child. When you implement these parental controls, you help to protect your child when they are doing the things they want and need to do online.

PARENTAL CONTROL:
ONLINE ACTIVITY REPORTS

Does your internet service provider help you to set up what are called online activity reports for your child when they are online? Parental controls are things you should consider using. They will help your child to stay safe when they are online and they definitely will help you to know what your child is up to when they are online. Although you may think you are spying on your child, you are ultimately just protecting them from all that is potentially lurking on the web that could threaten them.

What's An Activity Report?

A parental control activity report is put in place to help protect your child while they are online by informing you of what they are doing while they are there. It will provide you a report of what they've been doing when they are signed onto their account. This can help you know where they've gone and who they've talked to. Most importantly, it helps you to monitor if they are being safe online.

You may be able to learn many things from these reports. They will help you to know ho many emails they are getting as well as who they are getting them from and who they are sending them to. It will help you to know what websites they have visited including those that are the most frequently visited. Some activity reports will even help you to know what types of websites they have tried to visit but that are restricted through the use of your parental controls. This allows your child to stay protected while communicating with others online.

The activity report does not have to be something that you tell your child about, if you feel that you don't want to. It is a report that comes to the master account or the person responsible for the child's screen name account. The best thing is that your child can remain safe and you'll know about what potential risks they are taking and then be able to protect them from making mistakes. It is rare to be able to prevent mistakes that your child makes. Simply taking note of what they are doing will also help you to have some peace of mind when you can't watch over their shoulder when they are on the web.

PARENTAL CONTROL THROUGH WEBSITE BROWSING

Your child came home from school today talking about a website that they just have to visit. Parental controls allow you to provide your child with the protection they need when online and visiting websites that they learn about. If you are a parent that isn't sure about the type of protection that this software can provide in regards to website browsing, it pays to learn more about it. In fact, you may want to invest some time in learning what options are out there.

Each parental control software that are available offers different types of protection and different levels of it. Yet, as you may know, these elements are in place with your guidance. You'll need to make the decisions about what is right for your child and what is not. When it comes to web browsing, you can limit as much as you want or as little as you want them to access.

The highest level of access in regards to web browsing with parental controls does not allow for any website access. Move up a step and the child is able to visit only websites that you deem are okay and approve. Next step up usually allows your child to visit kid based websites that are known to be safe locations on the web. Finally, you can give them full access to online web browsing without any restrictions, if you like.

You should set the website browsing abilities on your parental control software to fit your child's age and their ability to navigate the web. Each child is different here, but you can base the information on what they like to do and what you want to protect them from. Select the level of protection that's appropriate for your child then enforce it with your internet service provider's parental controls.

PARENTAL CONTROL AND CHAT

Many kids enjoy getting on the web to talk to their friends. Parental controls can help you to protect them in these situations. You may ask why they can't just pick up the phone and call their friend. Or, you may wonder what is so great about typing in their responses to friends. Regardless of why online chatting is so much fun, children are doing it more and more and at younger ages. So, how can you protect your child from entering the wrong chat room? And, can you know what they are talking about there?

Chat rooms are the most common type of communication tool after instant messaging. In these cases, the individual visits a specific website that has a chat room. In these rooms, people come together from all areas of the world or just specific areas, depending on the type of room that it is. This is also one of the prime locations for a predator to pretend to be a child and therefore come into contact with your child.

With parental controls, you can adjust your child's ability to communicate in chat rooms. You can completely restrict them from all chat rooms, allow them access to some chat rooms that you approve or keep them only in kid friendly chat rooms that the software has approved. Each of these options are yours to consider. You have to determine what the right level of protection is available to you.

Parental controls usually can monitor where your child is going and attempting to go with the use of activity reports. But, they may not be able to tell you what's going on in the chat room. There are other software tools that you can purchase and use discretely to monitor this information, if you would like to. With some parental control over the chat room, you will feel better about your child being online.

PARENTAL CONTROL AND EMAIL

Email is something that kids use all of the time. Parental controls offer you some way to help protect your child from these experiences. Through the use of parental control ability, you can keep your child as well as your online computer network, safe from the spam and inappropriate email that could potentially come through to them while they are on the web. All parental control software is different, to some degree, but all can provide you with the ability to protect your child in regards to email.

Email modifications can be set up for each child that has their own screen name. In fact, giving them a screen name gives them an email account. On the youngest of internet users there may be no need to allow them to use email. But, as a child gets older, email becomes a standard part of the online experience and therefore is something that they really want to take advantage of. It is up to you to allow or not to allow email communications and parental control software will help you to make the decision as to what to include.

Email protection can be completely restricted, limited by only those you approve to communicate with your child through email, or it can be something you use spam filters on. If you use spam filters on your child's email account, you'll need to adjust the setting to the appropriate level (many times the highest filtration) to protect them from the elements there.

There is no doubt that you will need to use some type of parental control to monitor your child's email capabilities. Predators can use email as a way to come into contact with your child. It also is a large vulnerability to your computer in regards to spyware and spam. Therefore, you should select the appropriate level of protection for your child's email.

PARENTAL CONTROL AND INSTANT MESSAGING

Probably the most vulnerable area of the online experience to your child happens to be one of the most used tools by them. That is instant messaging. Parental controls may be able to provide you with the help you need in regards to these needs, though. Instant messaging is fun and cool. Kids love the fact that they can get online and talk with their friends. It is also an affordable way to communicate, being free of charge, for long distance conversations. Yes, the phone is still going to be used and yes there are plenty of times when you'll wonder about the fascination with instant messaging, but nevertheless, you'll need parental controls for it.

When it comes to parental controls for instant messaging, there are many different ways that protection can be used. The most commonly used is with an approval list. You get to choose the people that your child can communicate with by monitoring their list of friends. If they have someone new they would like to talk with, they have to have approval from the master screen name to do that. This means that you know exactly who they are chatting with.

One of the most important things to remember about instant messaging is that there are many different services available. Many computer systems actually have several installed on the computer already, even if you have never used them. That means that a crafty child can open these software tools, set them up and use them, without you even knowing that they are doing so and going completely around parental controls in the process.

For this reason, as well as overall protection, you should monitor how they are using instant messaging services and make sure that the parental control tools that you use monitor all internet access methods not just those that are through your internet service provider. This will give you the best control over your child while they are online.

"BECAUSE" JUST ISN'T THE ANSWER

Children are inquisitive by nature. When they are younger, it's usually because they want to better understand something. When they are older, it's because they want to better understand why you think something is important and why they should also feel the same way. Regardless of their age, it's imperative that when setting forth the rules and expectations in your home, your child understands there is no room for questioning the rules you set forth and the consequences of breaking the rules.

Younger children usually do not understand a lengthy explanation of why it's important that they be home from their friend's home at a certain time or why they aren't allowed to play ball in the house. But the one thing they do strive to do most of the time is to make their parents proud and happy. So when a young child asks "Why?" or "Why not?" when they are told they can't play with something or someone or why they have to obey a rule you've set forth, simply explain to them that "because it makes me happy when you follow the house rules and do what I have asked of you." You should avoid using the term, "Because I said so," as that only adds to the child's frustration and confusion.

Older children, adolescents and teenagers alike will probably require more from your explanation. When they question "Why?" or "Why not?" it's best to directly, honestly and clearly state your reasoning. "I asked you to be home by 10 p.m. because we have to be at the dentist's office first thing in the morning for your check-up and we can't be late." It is also a great opportunity for you to reiterate the consequences of breaking the rule. "If you are not home by 10 p.m., you'll be grounded from going to your friend's house for a week." Be consistent, be firm, and be clear.

Though your child may challenge you by asking your reasoning why a rule has been put in place, it also shows their growth as an individual thinker. So try not to get angry or frustrated when they do so; realize it's their way of understanding their world around them.

ENCOURAGE YOUR CHILD TO FEEL IMPORTANT

It's imperative for a child's healthy development to feel important and worthy. Healthy self- esteem is a child's armor against the challenges of the world. Kids who feel good about themselves seem to have an easier time handling conflicts and resisting negative pressures. They tend to smile more readily and enjoy life. These kids are realistic and generally optimistic. It's also been shown that children who feel important are well-rounded, respectful, and excel in academics, extracurricular activities and hobbies and develop healthy relationships with their peers.

In contrast, for children who do not feel important or cherished have low self-esteem, and challenges can become sources of major anxiety and frustration. Children who think poorly of themselves have a hard time finding solving problems, and may become passive, withdrawn, or depressed.

You are the biggest influence in your child feeling important, valued and worthy. Remember to praise your child for a job well done, and also for putting for a valiant effort. Praise the good traits they naturally possess, and help them find ways to learn from their mistakes and failures. Be honest and sincere in your praise. Help them realize that you also suffer from self doubt and can make mistakes from time to time, but that you know that you are important, valued and loved. When you nurture your own self -esteem and importance, your child will learn to do the same, so be sure to lead by example and steer clear of self-depreciating yourself or engaging in activities that lower your self-worth or importance.

Your child may have inaccurate or irrational beliefs about themselves, their abilities or their traits. Accentuate the positive about your child, and encourage your child to set realistic expectations and standards for themselves. Help them identify traits or skills they'd like to improve and help them come up with a game plan for accomplishing that goal. Encourage your child to become involved in cooperative activities that foster a sense of teamwork and accomplishment.

Through these and other positive, affirming activities, your child is sure to develop a strong sense of self importance, value and worth which will carry into their adult years.

44

FOLLOW THROUGH IS THE KEY
TO SUCCESSFUL DISCIPLINE

Let's face it. There are just some days when it would just seem easier to let your child have his way than feeling like you're fighting a losing battle when trying to discipline them. They beg, plead, cry, barter and scream - anything to get out of doing the time for their crime. However, don't lose your strength and your will during this time. It's times like these when consistent disciplinary action is imperative to teaching your child positive and acceptable behaviors. There is no room for negotiation when it comes to bad behaviors and there should be no room for exceptions when it comes time for punishing misdeeds or bad behavior.

Hopefully before any misdeeds occur, you've sat down with your child and discussed the consequences of misdeeds and inappropriate behavior or decisions. Be concise and consistent when discussing these consequences so that when the time to

45

implement them comes, you can follow through with ease. Children are classically testing the boundaries and limits set on them on a continual basis, and the temptation to 'bend the rules' just once or twice can be overwhelming when they're really trying your patience. But be firm yet fair. Emphasize that this was the understood consequence for this particular misdeed or inappropriate action, and that now is not the time to negotiate. Afterwards, take time out to discuss the situation with your child, and if it seems that perhaps a consequence that worked at first isn't working anymore, rethink that punishment and negotiate with your child. Of course, parameters that are set for their well-being or safety should never be negotiated. But in other instances, it may be time to develop a new consequence based on your child's age, temperament or maturity level.

It's also imperative that your spouse and any other adult caregivers are all on the same page and following through on punishments with the same level of consistency and clarity. Should you determine that what was once working isn't working anymore and develop a new parameter, be sure all adult caregivers are brought into the loop so that follow through remains consistent and clear.

PARENTING - WHEN A CHILD ASKS WHY

Children, by nature, are inquisitive. While young, they question because they want a better understanding of something. When they become older, they question because they want a better understanding of why they must give importance to the same things that you do.

Irrespective of how old the child is, it is important that when you are making the expectations and rules, the child does not question the validity of your claim and fully understands the consequences of disobedience.

Children of a younger age, do not usually understand the entire reason behind why it is necessary for them to be back home from a friends place at a particular time or why, while in the house, they shouldn't play ball. But to their credit, they always strive to make their parents happy and proud. This is why, whenever a child asks 'why not' or 'why' when they are told to go to bed early or to do some chores, you should never say 'because I say so'. Instead tell them that they should do it because it makes you happy when he or she follows the rules that have been set and does what you have asked. Giving no explanation or just making a demand adds to the child's confusion and frustration.

Teenagers, adolescents and older children will perhaps require a more elaborate explanation. Their why's and why not's should be met with a clearly comprehensive reason. " I do not want you to stay out till after 10 because we have to be at the airport early in the morning and I don't want us to be late." This will also be a good time to reiterate what happens on breaking a rule. " if you are not back by 10, you will be grounded for a week". You should exercise clarity, consistency and firmness.

Although a child may constantly question the requirement of putting a rule and the irrelevancy of it, it also shows that the child is growing to be an individual thinker. Therefore it is best you do not get frustrated or angry at them when they question you; remember it is their own method of understanding the world.

ENCOURAGE YOUR CHILD
TO FEEL IMPORTANT

If a child must develop in a healthy manner, it is necessary that he feels worthy and important. A good self-esteem is a child's safety against a world of challenges. When you feel good about yourself, you find it easier to handle challenges and conflicts and resist negative pressure. Such children tend to readily smile and mostly enjoy their lives. They are optimistic and realistic.

Children with a healthy self-esteem are proven to be over all respectful and well-rounded kids who usually do well in academics as well as extra-curricular activities and have a healthy relationship with their friends and peers.

On the other hand, children who have a damaged sense of self worth have lower self-esteem and they are not able to cope up with challenges and are often anxious and frustrated. It is common for children with low self-esteem to show withdrawal symptoms as they get more depressed and passive and show weak problem solving ability.

Parents are instrumental in how their children feel about themselves and it is their duty to make sure their children feel worthy and loved. When you child does a good job, remember to always praise him or her for the job as well as for the effort. Recognize and compliment their natural traits and support them in the process of learning from failures and mistakes. You should always be sincere and honest when you praise them. They must learn that everybody suffers self-doubt in their lives but regardless of how often you make mistakes, it is important to feel valued and important. When you teach by example and show your child how you go about dealing positively with day-to-day matters, the child automatically learns the same. Never expose the child to a self-depreciating environment or activities that lower your own worth.

Often children have irrational and inaccurate beliefs about themselves and their traits and abilities. Emphasize your child's positive qualities and urge them to have realistic expectations and to set proper standards for themselves. Encourage them to recognize their positive traits and skills and show them how to develop these so that they can accomplish their goals. Also to ensure that your child has good team spirit, encourage involvement in cooperative activities.

Giving your child a positive environment with positive activities ensures that your child will develop a strong self esteem and a high sense of worth and value which will equip them in their adult years.

FOLLOW THROUGH IS THE KEY
TO SUCCESSFUL DISCIPLINE

The truth is, that sometimes we feel it is much simpler just letting your child get away with something than fighting a battle you are anyway going to lose. They just make you give up by pleading, screaming, begging and crying that you just don't have the heart or patience any more to go through with your point. However, you must not lose your will or your strength at such times. Its at these times that disciplinary action is necessary so that your child learns acceptable and positive behavior. Bad behavior should not be made negotiable and there shouldn't be any scope for exceptions in terms of punishment for misbehavior and bad deeds.

Hopefully, before the occurrence of any misdeeds, you would have discussed and explained to your child the consequences of inappropriate behavior and misdeeds. They should understand clearly what action will be taken for bad behavior. Be clear, concise and consistent in explaining these so that when it comes to implementation, you can follow through easily. Children tend to test the limits and boundaries that are set for them and it is easy to let them bend the rule when your patience wanes. But you must be firm and fair and without loosing your ground explain that this was the consequence discussed and so it shall be. But do not forget to discuss the issue with the child and work out a better solution if the question of one arises. But you need to constantly consider your child's age and maturity and accordingly work out disciplinary action.

Sometimes as a child grows, so should the way we approach them.

It is necessary that your spouse as well any other caregiver, are in agreement with you and follow through with the same consistency and clarity when it comes to punishments. If you decide to make some changes in this area, make sure that all the other adults involved are informed so that the follow through always remains clear and consistent.

MAKE QUALITY TIME WITH
YOUR CHILD COUNT

Today, we all have such busy lives, what with the household chores, social activities and work; we hardly get to spend any time with our children. But as you know, spending quality time with your children is one of the most important things in bringing them up. It is through this that the bond between child and parent is strengthened, and the child begins to count on you and trust you. Parents who spend enough time with their children find that their child is doing better in school, hobbies and sports. Though you can schedule the time you spend with your child, spontaneity is always the best option. Therefore, it is best you spend time with your children in a relaxed environment and that you do things that you can both enjoy.

You might be wondering where you will find that kind of time. But you need to prioritize and dig out enough time from your busy schedule. Here is a list of things you could do with your child to make the most of the time you have available.

Go through the list of household chores and see which you can leave out or spend lesser time on in order to spare some time. You can also keep some chores for after your child's bedtime so that you can spend that time with your child.

You can even make some of your routines together interesting. You can sing songs together on your way to day care. You can even use the time spent in the car while driving to and from school to discuss things going on in your child's life.

When you have two or more children, it is important to give each individual attention. It might be difficult for you and you might really have to try very hard, but make sure you are creative and flexible while spending time with each child. And at no cost should you cancel out on time spent with each child. If you do this, the child may feel that he or she is less important than the grocery shopping or the dry cleaning.

Children need routine and stability, so ensure that the quality time you plan takes place regularly. You can use weekend mornings to take the dog for a walk together, or you can choose one day per week to have an eat out. There are many ways of spending time together, just make sure that it counts.

OUR EVER-CHANGING ROLE AS A PARENT

Our children grow up even before we realize it. It seems like just yesterday that they were crawling around trying to walk and suddenly they're in school, making friends, learning new things and becoming independent. It has been said that as soon as children are born, they are learning to let go. Accordingly, our strategies of parenting must change. Our parenting role must adapt the growth and change that our children go through, maturing and developing with them.

As a child grows, so does their temperament and personality which is unique to them. Without knowing, you would have developed parenting skills that cater to the individuality of your child. No two people are exactly and completely alike, and this applies for children as well. This should reflect in your parenting. Certain children are less sure of themselves and need more guidance while others are very fast at learning and might not require you to constantly guide them. We must according to the child's requirement and need, guide the child and give him or her encouragement to become more independent. While encouraging an independent attitude you must also teach them that it is not wrong to ask for help when required and we must praise and compliment their good deeds, traits and actions.

Our ears and eyes are the most reliable tools we posses in order to adjust and assess our parenting skills. We must keep open eyes and ears to see and hear what is happening in our children's lives and what they are trying to tell us. We must be available to our children whenever they need us as well as constantly urge them to be strong and independent.

Sometimes it depends on the situation. A child may not necessarily require you to be directly involved in their academic progress but might require your support when it comes to social issues like making friends and talking to new people.

The bottom line is that your parenting skills should grow and mature your child does. Keep an open ear and eye to communicate openly and honestly with your children, and you will both mature into great individuals.

POSITIVE DISCIPLINE WITHOUT
HURTING YOUR CHILD

Children, very often, try our patience and we end up losing our temper and calm. It is very easy to end up feeling annoyed, sad, angry, irritated, hurt and confused. These periods of time are the true test of our parenting skills. Therefore it becomes important that we exercise discipline firmly but kindly. And the truth is, nobody wants to hurt their children either physically or verbally. When we feel that what our child has done is wrong and we want to teach him or her this distinction, yelling, hitting and punishing the child is the worst course of action to take.

When teaching our children discipline, our goal should be to teach them what cooperative, kind, respectful and responsible behavior is. The best method of teaching this is to be consistent, ensuring that the same punishment follows through for the same misbehavior, and to explain the discipline honestly and openly with the child afterwards.

While enforcing disciplinary action, the temperament, age and maturity level must always be kept in mind. Disciplinary actions should always be discussed well in advance so that the child, when confronted with a particular kind of situation, is fully aware of the consequences, and hopefully chooses to behave accordingly. And most significantly, you must never forget that it is the child's behavior in a certain instance that you disapprove of and not the child itself.

If required, you can give yourself a little time before deciding to respond to a misdeed of your child. Sometimes we need a little time to cool off before dealing with the child in order to think carefully and not make any mistakes of our own. Hitting and yelling should be strictly avoided.

As a parent, you must keep your mind open, and should be willing to learn from and with your child. Every human makes mistakes and we must keep in mind that every disciplinary action may not work for every child. Children are as unique as anybody else, sometimes more so, and it is important that any form of discipline enforced on the child is made fitting to his or her character and individual needs of the child and parents. With enough love, patience, forethought, understanding and firmness, the process of discipline will have a positive outcome.

PROTECT YOUR CHILD'S EMOTIONAL WELL-BEING

So often do we get caught up in the rigmarole of our hectic and busy lives with our jobs and our families, that we easily forget one of the most important aspects of our child's life - his or her emotional well-being. The most critical times in a child's life are the first three years. In this critical phase, constantly switching providers of childcare or having a 'part time' parent come irregularly in their lives can be extremely destabilizing and traumatic for the child. Just as the child's physical needs are met, it is equally important to meet his or her emotional needs and it is the duty of the involved adults like parents, educators and care providers to make a joint effort towards achieving this on a daily basis. If a child's emotional requirements are not satisfied, especially up till the age of three, it can have devastating effects on him or her. It can result in disruptive, defiant and violent behavior.

There are a number of reasons why the first three years of the child's life are so important. This is the period when emotional separation and bonding takes place. Misbehavior on the child's part can result if either one of these processes is interrupted. This can have far reaching consequences in their relationships in life and can hinder the development of healthy relationships when they become adolescents and adults.

The brain undergoes extremely rapid development up till the age of three; a kind of development which never repeats again in life. By the age of three, the child's brain has already cemented from what they have experienced up till that point. Therefore, it becomes necessary that these experiences should be supportive, loving, positive and safe, so that the brain can be conditioned to function positively. If they have had hurtful, frightening, dangerous or abusive experiences, then without doubt the brain will be conditioned to expect negativity.

For all these reasons, it is imperative that the caregivers, parents and all involved adults should try hard to ensure that emotionally, the child's needs are always met positively and in a manner that is healthy and constructive. Parents should make sure that the care providers of the child are consistent and stable and see to it that the care provider is not changed too many times. The child will feel secure and safe only if it is given a consistent and structured routine and schedule. During this period, you must try to spend a lot of quality time with your child regardless of how busy and stressed you may be. Sensing stress is a frightful situation for children and you must ensure this doesn't take place. Therefore you need to constantly remind him or her that you are not too busy to take him or her out.

You must never forget that a child's emotional need is as important as its physical needs and you need to do your part in order to ensure that your child knows he or she is secure, safe, loved and treasured.

SUCCESSFUL TWO-WAY COMMUNICATIONS WITH YOUR CHILD

Communicating effectively with one's child is perhaps one of the toughest challenges that parents have to face. In spite of trying to open a two-way communication line with our child, it gets frustrating if we find that their attention is not on the ongoing conversation or on us at all. We complain about broken communication lines when all the time we find it completely alright to converse with them when we are folding clothes, reading the newspaper, writing letters or cooking meals.

By nature children get easily distracted and do not always respond as expected to their environment. It becomes the duty of the parents to encourage positive communication patterns and to discourage the act of ignoring communication. In order to make sure that a non-verbal agreement does not ensue, it is important to educate the child on proper communication forms and hence prevent this. Teaching by example is the best method. While conversing, you must direct your complete attention on them and total focus on the conversation. Allow voicemail to take your calls, turn the television off or go to a room with no distractions if that's what it takes.

You must gently and in age appropriate terms explain to your child what is wrong with their form of communication and why it doesn't work. Even when there are hard questions, you must show you child the most effective manner of communication. Become a good listener. You must encourage them to tell their side of the story and to voice their opinions and respond positively to show that you understand their point of view.

You must communicate with your child in a consistent manner. You must send out the same signals ach time you interact. The child must be allowed to see that you will definitely call their attention whenever unwanted behavior takes place.

Kids are after all kids and it is normal for them to be non-communicative and non-reactive sometimes. Your child is your domain and you should know best how to interpret his or her behavior and gauge improvement in communication skills. Modeling positive communication skills is the best way of ensuring that your child imbibes healthy communication patterns.

THE TRUTH ABOUT LYING

Honesty and dishonesty are qualities that a child learns at home. Often parents are perturbed when their child lies.

It is common for young children to tell tall tales and make up stories. This is a normal tendency as kids enjoy telling and hearing stories that are fun. Children often tend to confuse the difference between fantasy and reality. This is perhaps more as a result of an extremely active imagination than of an attempt to hide the truth. As children get older, they may tell lies to suite their needs, like shirking responsibility and avoiding work. Parents should treat each instance of lying as an isolated one and respond by teaching the child about the necessity of trust and honesty.

Sometimes adolescents feel that it is alright to lie in certain situations like not telling ones girlfriend or boyfriend the real reason for a breakup as they are afraid of hurting someone else's feelings. Adolescents might also lie to retain a sense of privacy and feel psychologically independent of their parents. The main role models in a child's life are his or her parents. When parents catch their child lying, they should approach the matter gently but firmly, emphasizing the difference between a lie and the truth and the necessity for honesty. They should try to communicate to their child and find out the reason for dishonesty and help the child find an alternative. It is best to lead by example and a parent should never lie, and if they do, emphasize the inappropriateness of it. Consequences of lying must be discussed clearly and in a comprehensive manner with the child early in his or her life. There are, however, some forms of dishonesty that should cause concern and might be a symptom of some underlying emotional problem. Sometimes children know the difference between a lie and the truth but choose to make up elaborate stories to gain attention.

Other adolescents or children, who seem to be sensible, can also fall prey to repetitive lying. It is common for them to feel that a lie is the most convenient method of dealing with the expectations of teachers, parents and friends. Here the child is not trying to be malicious or bad but just falls into a habit of repetitive lying. If the repetitive lying goes beyond a point, it is best to take it seriously and consult a professional child or adolescent psychologist who can provide help in time.

TRAINING THE FUSSY EATER

When it comes to eating, toddlers can be extremely fussy, rejecting new food half of the time. Most of the toddlers are like this and it is no surprise that food issues cause a lot of anxiety in parents.

Problems such as eating disorders and obesity can be avoided if healthy eating patterns are established early in life. There are many ways of ensuring your child consumes a variety of foods. You may even need to offer a certain type of food to your child at least 10 times before they finally agree to eat it. Many parents, unfortunately, give into frustration and give up after four or five tries.

You must make the food fun for the child. You can offer your growing toddler colorful foods such as raisins, carrot sticks, grapes, apples, crackers and cheese sticks which he or she will find fun and interesting. You must explain to them in their language how good food can help them play longer and run faster by making them bigger and stronger.

Parents are usually the children's role models and children try to emulate them. If you eat only a certain kind of food, your child will learn to have a restricted taste too. Don't let your preferences put a limit on your child's food intake. It is possible that yours and your child's taste vary and you might be serving them an item that they simply don't like. Always openly eat a wide variety of foods in front of your children so they might try to do the same.

If you have a healthy and energetic child, then they must be eating well. If you still feel unsure, keep watch over what and how much food they consume over the day. Unlike adults, children eat often and not just three meals per day. Snacks and handfuls can add up to quite a bit. To confirm, you can take your child to a pediatrician and check your child's weight and height status.

Don't worry too much because a child will always eat, unless he or she is ill. They have very good judgment when it comes to hunger and fullness. Always be calm and patient during meal times and ensure your child has access to a fair variety of foods. You never know, you and toddler may find something in common.

OUR EVER-CHANGING ROLE AS A PARENT

We watch our children grow right before our very eyes. It seems like yesterday they were a baby learning to crawl, walk, and feed themselves, and now they're in school, involved in activities, making friends, and learning to be more and more independent. Parents before us have said that from the time they're born, we are constantly learning to let go. As a result, our parenting strategies have to change. As our child grows, develops, learns, and matures, so does our parenting role.

As your child has grown, you undoubtedly have discovered they have their own unique personality and temperament. You've probably unconsciously redeveloped your parenting skills around the individual needs of your child. And no two children are exactly alike, and therefore, neither should your parenting style. Some children may need more guidance and feel more unsure of themselves, so we've become used to having to guide, lead, show and encourage that child consistently through their childhood while still trying to encourage independence and give praise in order to build their self esteem and confidence level. Yet another child may be very intrinsically motivated and very willful and not need a great deal of guidance or leadership from you. While you encourage their independence, it's also important that you also encourage their ability to ask for help when needed and continue to praise good deeds, actions, and traits.

The most important tools we have in order to successfully adjust our parenting skills are our eyes and our ears. We have to see what's going on with our child and we have to hear what they are telling us. It's important that we encourage our child to be their own individual while still being available to them at whatever level or degree they need us to be. Sometimes it's situation-specific as well. A child may not need us to be as directly involved with their schooling to ensure their overall academic success, but they may need us to be more involved in their social life as they may be feeling a bit shaky or scared when it comes to making new friends or meeting new people.

So the bottom line is this: as your child grows and changes, so should your parenting skills. Keep your eyes and ears open and communicate honestly and openly with your child, and you'll both mature gracefully.

Printed by Libri Plureos GmbH in Hamburg,
Germany